Toilet Training, Bedwetting and Soiling

by
Martin Herbert

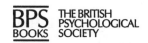
BPS BOOKS
THE BRITISH
PSYCHOLOGICAL
SOCIETY

First published in 1996 by BPS Books (The British Psychological Society), St Andrews House, 48 Princess Road East, Leicester LE1 7DR, UK.

A catalogue record for this book is available from the British Library.

ISBN 1 85433 186 8

Typeset by Ralph Footring, Derby.

Printed in Great Britain by Stanley L. Hunt Printers Ltd., Rushden, Northants.

Contents

Toilet training, bedwetting and soiling

Introduction

Aims

This guide is for use by those people who work with parents and children, notably community practitioners such as school nurses, health visitors, social workers and community medical officers who may be asked by worried parents when, how, and even whether, to potty train their children. It is also for those practitioners and trainees in the health and social services who are faced with even more worried parents whose children have been unsuccessful in learning bowel and/or bladder control, or have lost those skills.

The approach to this work is based on the *collaborative model*. This is my preferred way of carrying out therapy or training because of the evidence that a partnership with parents in the 'therapeutic' endeavour is not only more effective with behaviour problems and difficulties such as incontinence than the expert model, but also more acceptable to parents and to the child (Webster-Stratton and Herbert, 1994).

This is an introductory, which is to say *basic,* text, and it should be used in association with additional instruction such as workshops and lectures in the case of the novice and as a source of information and further reading for supervised practice. The need for medical checks, where appropriate, is emphasized throughout the text.

Objectives

After studying the guide you should be able to answer parents'/caregivers' questions about toilet-training, and the following three key clinical questions about bedwetting (enuresis) and soiling (encopresis):

1. What is bedwetting/soiling and what are its ramifications?

2. Why do children fail to become continent or lose the skill after initial success?

3.   How do I help a child to stop bedwetting and/or soiling: or better still, how do I help the parents and child to help themselves?

More specifically, you should be able to:

> describe and recognize (diagnose) enuresis and encopresis and their various manifestations;

> carry out an assessment of salient features: physical, psychological, social and emotional;

> formulate the causal patterns for incontinence problems in a *general* sense and the determinants of a *particular* case referred to you;

> know whether, or when, to refer the child to an appropriate specialist for initial additional assessments (for example, medical) and/or treatment (for example, psychotherapeutic);

> plan, initiate and follow up a training programme (a behavioural programme based on social learning theory) to eliminate soiling.

Part I: Potty training

'Potty training' is the phrase commonly used to describe the steps parents take in helping children to develop bowel and bladder control (a physical achievement) and teaching them where to put faeces and urine (a social skill). Potty training is one of the most significant developmental tasks of toddlerhood. Dollard and Miller (1950) put it this way:

> Within a relatively short space of time the toddler must learn, under pain of losing his/her mother's esteem, to attach anxiety to all the cues produced by excretory materials, to their sight, smell and touch . . . to deposit faeces and urine only in a prescribed and secret place, and to clean its body. It must later learn to suppress unnecessary verbal reference to these matters.

Control of the bowels is attained before bladder control and the developmental sequence is *generally* as follows:

Stage 1 – Bowel control *at night*.
Stage 2 – Bowel control *during the day*.
Stage 3 – Bladder control *during the day*.
Stage 4 – Bladder control *at night*.

The sequence may vary for individual children: some achieve bowel and bladder control simultaneously, and girls tend to be quicker than boys in becoming continent.

A child might be considered 'potty trained' when s/he is able to use the toilet (or potty) reasonably independently, perhaps with assistance over bottom-wiping and clothing. Many parents make the issue of toilet training a rod for their own backs by trying too hard, too soon or too late and warfare with the toddler breaks out. Knowledge of the 'norms' (what to expect in normal development), especially the wide range of individual differences, should help parents to feel a bit less hurried and more relaxed about this teaching task.

Norms

The age at which control is achieved by children varies greatly between cultures and within our own culture, depending on parental expectations.

A study by Weir (1982) of 706 three-year-olds in an outer London borough produced the following results:

➤ 23 per cent of boys and 13 per cent of girls were wet by day (wetting more than once a week);

➤ 55 per cent of boys and 40 per cent of girls were wet by night.

➤ 21 per cent of boys and 11 per cent of girls were 'soilers' (that is, had soiled at least once during the previous month).

Norms for soiling

Most children have achieved bowel control by both day and night at between three and a half and four years of age, so four years is a realistic minimum age for judging whether there is a problem in bowel control (encopresis).

Norms for wetting

In some cultures bedwetting is not seen as a problem at all, and in others night-time dryness is seen as an important developmental task to be achieved as soon as possible. Every newborn comes into the world with an inability to control wetting; the young infant's development is such that when his/her bladder is full of urine, an automatic or reflex action occurs and the bladder empties regardless of the time of day or where the child is. As children get older they eventually gain control of their wetting so that they can 'hang on' when they have a full bladder, and delay wetting until they can get to the toilet. At the age of 5–7 years, 2 to 4 per cent of children wet during the day at least once a week, and approximately 8 per cent are wet at least monthly. For most children the control that they learn during the day transfers to the night; they learn to hold on for the whole night or to wake up when their bladder is full and take themselves to the toilet. There is no one age at which children cease to wet the bed, but there is a gradual decrease in the number of children who wet the bed; from every child at birth, to 1 or 2 in every 100 children at age 15 (see Table 1). Five years old is a realistic minimum age for judging there to be a problem in bladder control ('diurnal' or 'nocturnal enuresis').

James Anthony (1957) describes the complexities of the learning process for the child as follows:

> From the child's eye view, the toilet ritual, as practised by the adults of our compulsive communities, must sometimes appear as an exacting and complex ordeal far removed from the simple evacuations into the

Table 1   Frequency of bedwetting

Age in years	Approximate number of children in every 100 who wet the bed
2	75
3	40
4	30
5	20
6–9	12
10–12	5
by 15	1-2

nursery pot. It is his business with maternal prompting, to become aware of defecation cues in time, to stop his play in response to this, to suppress the desire for immediate excretion, to search for and find an appropriate place for the purpose, to ensure adequate privacy for himself, to unfasten his clothes, to establish himself securely on the toilet seat … to recognize an end-point to the proceedings, to cleanse himself satisfactorily, to flush the toilet, to refasten his clothes, to unbolt the door and emerge successfully to resume his interrupted play at the point where he left off.

Toileting skills

Toilet skills include the following:

➤ having words (e.g. wee/pooh) for urine and faeces, and for the places they are deposited in (e.g. potty, toilet);

➤ sitting on the toilet;

➤ going to the toilet (e.g. indicating need to caregiver, going unaided);

➤ managing clothing/wiping, when at toilet;

➤ having control (continence).

Dr Alison Tierney (1973) provides a breakdown of toileting skills. The development of each of these abilities can further be broken down usefully into stages or steps.

Continence

1.   Child uses toilet when placed on it and is incontinent at all other times.

2.   Child has established some regularity and uses toilet more frequently than is incontinent.
3.   Child urinates in toilet regularly and has only infrequent incontinent episodes.
4.   Child urinates only in the toilet and is otherwise continent.

Sitting

1.   Child is placed on toilet and is restrained to sit.
2.   Child is placed on toilet and sits unrestrained.
3.   Child is helped to sit on toilet and sits unrestrained.
4.   Child sits on toilet independently.

Dressing

1.   Child co-operates passively when clothing is removed.
2.   Child actively assists when clothing is removed.
3.   Child removes or actively attempts to remove some of his clothing.
4.   Child removes his clothing independently.

Going

1.   Child is taken to toilet.
2.   Child indicates need to urinate.
3.   Child asks to go to the toilet.
4.   Child goes to the toilet independently.

The order in which children achieve the different skills is, as we have seen (p. 4), variable, some learning quickly, others slowly and a very small number not at all. The early steps can be facilitated by:

➤   anticipating the child who is regular (sitting him/her on the potty at the expected time or when the telltale signs (e.g. a red face) are visible);

➤   making a sit-on-the-pot part of the morning routine (before dressing) and evening routines (at bedtime);

➤   praising success (and effort);

➤   gradually increasing the frequency of sessions on the potty (avoid force and overlong and boring 'sittings');

➤   encouraging the child to let caregivers know when s/he has urinated or passed a bowel motion. The awareness of *having* wet or soiled precedes the awareness of *impending* urination or bowel movement!

➤   eventually leaving off nappies;

➤   teaching the child to help (and eventually manage) putting on and taking off of pants;

➤   reminding the child to ask for the potty – this means having it handy as there may be a rush to sit him/her on it;

➤   making liberal use of praise and encouragement for trying and success; avoid criticism and punishment.

➤   moving on eventually to the toilet, adapted for his/her use. (A step may be needed to help them reach.)

When it comes to bladder and bowel training the explanations in the *Hints for Parents* at the back of the guide may be helpful.

Mechanisms of control

The control of elimination via the bowels and rectum (see *Hints for Parents No. 4*) means inhibiting processes which are, at first, completely involuntary. The baby's muscles must mature until they are strong enough and coordinated enough to hold back the waste products that are trying to emerge from his or her body. Of all the muscles in the trunk region, those which control the organs of elimination are the slowest to come under voluntary control.

The total time required to complete bowel training has been found to be less when it is initiated relatively late. Sears, Maccoby and Lewin (1957) were able to show that when mothers began bowel training before the child was five months old, nearly ten months (on average) was required for success. But when training was begun later (at 20 months or older) only about five months were required. Children whose toilet training was begun between 5 and 14 months or after 19 months, manifested fewest emotional reactions during training.

Children are expected to achieve satisfactory bladder control during the day by the time they start school. Parents and teachers may tolerate occasional lapses in the infant school, but thereafter, an incontinent child is likely to come under increasing social pressure. It is perhaps not surprising that some children do not learn bladder control as infants, or easily lose (especially when under stress) their ability to control the bladder at night. We should perhaps be surprised that so many *do* manage to learn such a complicated skill. It is likely that unpleasant experiences involving stress make the learning of bladder control (as with other skills) more difficult.

The ability to stay dry at night usually occurs *after* learning to stay dry during the day. Nearly 70 per cent have that skill at three years of age, but some children do not begin to develop night-time control until after their third birthday, so there is no need to worry at an earlier stage if a child is somewhat slow to achieve success.

Children with learning difficulties

Almost all studies since the 1960s of daytime toilet training for children (and adults) with learning difficulties have been conducted within an *operant* (reward programme) or *stimulus–response* (classical conditioning) framework (see Smith and Smith, 1987). These methods have been demonstrated to be effective. However, when clients are being treated within a residential establishment, attention must be paid to factors other than the specific programme; for example, staff attitudes, toileting facilities, and so on. The backward chaining programme (see following) may prove useful, or, indeed, the routine training programme described in *Appendix 1*.

Smearing

Children who are intellectually challenged sometimes smear faeces, to the consternation of caregivers (and indeed, some children who do not have learning difficulties smear their faeces on walls or other places). Smearing can be caused by some of the same reasons as soiling. In addition, children who smear:

➤ might like playing with messy things;
➤ might be at the age when they learn about the body and be a bit too eager to 'experiment';
➤ may think it is bad to pass a motion, and try to hide it. Others put their hand to their pants to check if they have soiled, then wipe their dirty hands on the furniture;
➤ may simply not know at first that it is inappropriate to smear. Parents' reaction to it might teach them that they get attention for this, either positive or negative, and any attention may be better than no attention;
➤ may have emotional problems which require assessment.

Backward chaining

This method of training may be helpful with slow learners, as it breaks down the skill of toileting into small steps, the links in a chain. Instead of beginning at the beginning, one begins at the end of the chain of skills, with an analysis of the skills that are necessary for independent toileting. The use of backward chaining necessitates determining which of the necessary skills the child has. This determines where you start the programme.

The chain

The stages in backward chaining are as follow.

➤   Becoming aware, accurately, of the rectal sensations due to distension by faecal material.
➤   Entering the toilet.
➤   Preparing clothing for defecation.
➤   Controlling the motor elements of sphincter activity.
➤   Cleaning the body.
➤   Dressing.

Because it is more difficult to teach the first step of interpreting rectal sensations due to distension by faecal material than it is to teach the child to dress after toileting, start at the end of this chain and work backwards. Thus:

(a)   the child progressively masters the skills necessary for independent toileting;
(b)   the child gradually adds to the skills already learned, and consolidates them, by always ending with a skill that has been mastered.

Note

If the child has no toileting skills you start *at the end of the chain of necessary skills*, by teaching the child to dress after toileting. Once this has been mastered, move back a step to teaching the child to clean him/herself. Once cleaning and dressing are established, the child should be helped to acquire the necessary motor control for defecation, and so on, back through the chain. If backward chaining is combined with a reward system, reward the target behaviour and not the bowel movement. For example, at the first stage of the example given, the child should be rewarded for successful dressing, regardless of whether a bowel movement was produced. The reward should shift with the target behaviour, for example, from dressing to cleaning.

Part II: Enuresis

Whether a child has been wet all his/her life, or has more recently lost control of his/her bladder, s/he needs special help in the difficult task of learning bladder control. (This applies to children *over the age of five* – the age at which the majority might be expected to be continent at night). Nocturnal enuresis is usually defined as repeated involuntary passage of urine during sleep in the absence of any identified physical abnormality in children aged above five. The child will usually (and preferably) be examined first by a doctor in case there is a physical cause for the bedwetting, although organic aetiology (that is, physical or medical causation) is somewhat uncommon. When a child wets the bed, it seems that his/her brain is not properly aware of the amount of urine in the bladder, allowing it to empty automatically while s/he is sleeping.

Prevalence

The likelihood that a child will become continent spontaneously over a 12-month period is reduced sharply after the age of four (Shaffer, 1994). Nocturnal bedwetting at least once a week occurs in approximately 13 per cent (boys) or 14 per cent (girls) of five-year-olds (Rutter, Tizard and Whitmore, 1970), while some estimates (see Table 1) make the rate higher! The prevalence rate is 1 per cent to 2 per cent for youngsters over fifteen and for adults. Enuresis is a very common occurrence amongst children in residential establishments, and in many cases continues, if untreated, into late adolescence or even adulthood. Daytime wetting (diurnal enuresis) is present in approximately one in ten nocturnal enuretics. Bedwetting, as we have seen, is about equally common in boys and girls until five years of age; boys then predominate to the extent that by age eleven they are twice as likely to be wet as girls (Essen and Peckham, 1976).

Enuresis is not only a source of embarrassment to the sufferer, often invoking ridicule or punishment, but can place an intolerable burden upon family relationships, especially in large families living in overcrowded conditions, where several children may wet the bed.

For the majority of enuretics, to be a bedwetter carries adverse emotional consequences, and these children tend to exhibit some degree of reactive emotional disturbance.

Even when this is not apparently the case, enuresis imposes a limit on the child's choice of activities; few enuretics can happily go camping or stay with friends. In own-homes and residential establishments, the daily wash of bed linen is unpleasant and onerous; all too often both natural parents and house-parents are forced into a fatalistic acceptance of enuresis as an inevitable correlate of child upbringing.

Assessment

Primary enuresis. This problem represents a behavioural deficit. The child has never gained control of nocturnal wetting.

Secondary enuresis. Here the child reverts to bedwetting after a period of being dry. Onset is most common between the ages of 5 and 7 but uncommon after age 11. The child's control may, anyway, have been tenuous at best. As many as 25 per cent of preschoolers who have been continent for at least 6 months will start to wet again (Fergusson *et al.*, 1986). A period of stress may produce the regression.

A further distinction can also be made between children who are regularly and those who are intermittently enuretic.

Causation

The origins of nocturnal enuresis would seem to be multifactorial. Enuresis may have its origins in faulty learning. Because the peak age-range for the emergence of continence is between one-and-a-half and four-and-a-half years of age, it could be said that there is a 'sensitive' period for the emergence of night-time dryness. Harsh pressurizing of the child or (conversely) complacent neglect of training may lead to a failure of this development. Emotional problems are then superimposed when the child is made to feel acute shame at his or her 'babyish' ways. Only too often, as I have already mentioned, they have to endure punishment, scorn and ridicule at home and at school. Other contributory causal influences may be urological and medical factors, such as small functional bladder capacity, genetics, maturation and developmental disorders, and also a variety of psychological factors.

Physical causes

As many as ten per cent of all cases of enuresis are the result of medical (physical) conditions, most commonly urinary tract infections. Approximately one in twenty female and one in fifty male enuretics have such an infection. Other uncommon physical causes are chronic renal or kidney disease, diabetes, tumours and seizures. Such potentially important causes make an expert physical examination a matter of routine. Enuresis runs in families; some 70 per cent of clinically referred enuretics have a first-degree relative who was enuretic as a child.

Emotional influences (anxiety)

Children who wet the bed may also tend to be anxious or nervous children; what is not certain is the precise nature of the relationship between feeling anxious and wetting the bed.

A popular view is that anxiety is associated with bedwetting. This idea is supported by the fact that several studies have shown that after the successful treatment of bedwetting there is usually a decrease in anxiety and an improvement in the way the child feels about her/himself. This explanation seems plausible when we think about the problems of being a bedwetter. The child is often ridiculed by her/his brothers and sisters and may even be ridiculed by parents. Staying at a friend's house or going on school camps is not possible. It is even very difficult to hide the problem from neighbours, given the frequent appearance of sheets and blankets on the clothesline. It is not surprising that the bedwetter becomes very anxious about his/her problem.

Treatment

Over the years a number of methods have been suggested for the treatment of enuresis. Some of these have been based on scientific theory and research while others are merely 'old wives' tales'. A particularly common, but unsupported, belief is that bedwetting is related to depth of sleep – children wet the bed because they sleep deeply. Because of this unsupported idea, some parents in the past have implemented what could only be described as harsh regimes, for example making children sleep on hard beds to prevent deep sleep.

Medication

Many physicians turn to medication to treat their enuretic patients. A favourite drug is a tricyclic antidepressant, imipramine hydro-chloride (Tofranil). Certainly, an increase in urinary control tends to occur in about 25 to 40 per cent of cases in the first two weeks of treatment, but up to 95 per cent relapse following the withdrawal of medication. There is no clear theoretical rationale for the use of this drug. More sure, but more onerous and time-consuming, is the approach based on a training paradigm; treatment, in such cases, can be thought of as the teaching of new and more effective skills and more appropriate responses to stimuli.

Synthetic antidiuretics (e.g. desmopressin) have been used alone and in combination with the alarm system described below. The effects are comparable to those of the tricyclic antidepressants (Shaffer, 1994).

The enuresis alarm
(see *Hints for Parents No. 3* at the back of the guide)

The device known as the 'enuresis alarm' has been developed to help children (with the supervision of a professional) to overcome the problem of bedwetting. Basically, the alarm is made up of a pair of detector mats on the bed, connected to a buzzer next to the child's bed. As soon as the child begins to wet in her/his sleep, the buzzer sounds. The use of the alarm produces two actions – stopping the stream and waking – whenever the child's bladder begins to empty automatically during sleep.

Gradually the brain learns to connect these two actions with the feeling of a full bladder. After a time the brain becomes more aware of the amount of urine in the child's bladder, and begins itself to take the two actions of contracting the muscles and waking the child when the bladder is full. Eventually the child is able to sleep without wetting, waking up on his/her own if s/he needs to use the toilet at night.

Mini body (pants) alarm

Pants alarms for night-time and/or daytime toilet training are min-iature portable versions of the apparatus used in the treatment of bedwetting. A sensor is attached to the child's pyjama or underpants and the alarm is carried on a wrist band or in a pocket. The device delivers an auditory signal to the child (Schmidt, 1986).

Effectiveness

The evidence for the superiority of the alarm method (with rates of remission between 80 per cent and 90 per cent) over no-treatment and other-treatment control procedures is well documented for nocturnal enuresis (see Shaffer, 1994). While Doleys' (1977) data based on over 600 subjects revealed an average relapse rate of 40 per cent, nearly 60 per cent of those returned to continence after booster sessions.

Incentive systems

Because of the ease of producing some change in the child's motivation to be dry by offering rewards (reinforcement) for dryness, this is probably a good place to start for the parent of the bedwetter.

Rewards

One method is to provide a *special* reward for achieving a given (a *gradually* increasing) number of consecutive dry nights. The usual number of dry nights the child is expected to have to be considered 'trained' is fourteen in a row. If fourteen in a row are achieved the child is less likely to go back to wetting.

Star/sticker charts

Night (and day) wetting can sometimes be brought to an end by the use of a simple star or sticker chart for dry beds (or pants). When a negotiated number of stars is achieved, the child receives a special treat or privilege, or exchanges them for small items such as crayons, plasticine and so on at a fixed tariff. A record is kept on a chart (see *Appendix VII*) a little like a calendar, with a space for each day. Each time the child has a dry night a gold star (or colourful sticker) is placed in the appropriate place on the calendar and the child can see how well s/he is going by the number of stars on the chart. Sometimes this will be enough to motivate the child to be dry more often but can then be backed up by making sure that some other reward, such as an outing or TV viewing, is available only if a certain number of stars is earned each week. (For a colouring-in record of success, see *Appendix VI*.)

This method results in a marked reduction, and in some cases a cure, in up to 20 per cent of enuretics (Devlin and O'Cathain, 1990).

Encouraging and/or sanctioning

A child may continue to wet the bed because s/he is simply not motivated enough (or perhaps *encouraged* enough!) to learn to be dry. Indeed some instances have been observed where the child is able to wake up and go to the toilet when required but instead *chooses* to wet the bed. This is particularly likely to occur in the middle of winter, or if the route to the toilet is long and dark. Here it is important for parents to provide the necessary motivation for the child and to change the situation in some way so that going to the toilet and keeping the bed dry is more attractive than wetting the bed. However, there are problems associated with sanctioning/penalizing the child for wetting the bed as the problem may not be simply motivational and the child may be being punished unfairly. The punishment may lead to an increase in anxiety associated with wetting the bed.

A preferable alternative is to increase the child's desire to be dry and to make being dry a very attractive option. This means that the parent provides incentives for the child being dry and, at the same time, ignores those occasions on which the child wets. The easiest (and often most effective) strategy is to make sure that the child gets lots of praise and attention when a dry night is achieved.

Daytime (bladder-stretching) training

There is some evidence to suggest that bedwetters may have smaller bladder capacities than non-bedwetters. Training children to hold greater and greater amounts can increase the bladder capacity.

Daytime training involves having the child signal when s/he first feels the need to go to the toilet. S/he is then asked to hang on for five minutes before going. After five minutes are up s/he is told s/he can go and is praised extensively for his/her efforts. When the child can hold on easily for five minutes the length of time is gradually increased by five minute intervals, until the child can hang on for up to thirty minutes. This method helps her/him increase the capacity of the bladder so s/he can get through the night without having to go to the toilet.

This procedure certainly increases bladder capacity but its effectiveness in treating bedwetting has not been firmly established at this stage. It is a useful way of dealing with the problem of urgency of urination. (See *Appendix III: Daytime Record Sheet* at back of guide.)

Training the child to hold greater and greater quantities of fluid can increase bladder capacity. The child is encouraged to drink increased amounts of liquid and then hold back her/his need to urinate as long as possible. S/he is asked to urinate in a measuring cup and record how much s/he was able to hold. Each day the child tries to break her/his previous record and a reward is provided for success. (The bladder has a capacity of five to seven ounces on average in the six year old.)

The '*start and stop*' method while urinating (holding and letting go of the flow of urine) strengthens the muscles' and bladder valve's ability to inhibit urine flow.

Diurnal enuresis treatment programmes

The use of incentives for habit-training and portable body alarms also play their part in the treatment of daytime wetting (for example, Halliday *et al.*, 1987).

Part III: Encopresis

What is faecal soiling (encopresis)?

When stool enters the rectum, causing it to stretch, sensory nerves are stimulated. These nerves send a message to the brain telling us we are full and need to evacuate. However when the child withholds (for whatever reason) stool, his/her rectum enlarges slowly over weeks and months. Eventually it becomes so large that it can no longer be suddenly stretched by the passage of stool into the rectum. At this point the child no longer knows if his/her rectum is full or not. Because the appropriate messages are not getting through, a large, hard impaction of stool forms in the rectum and the constipation becomes so severe that it leads to a partial blockage of the bowel. Some of the motions liquefy and leak around the impacted area, soiling the child's underwear (see *Hints for Parents No. 5*). Children with encopresis due to rectal impaction cannot prevent themselves from soiling. They are unaware of their blockage and unable to prevent the leakage.

To summarize, the soiling occurs because the child has lost the normal anal reflex through excessive constipation and subsequent dilation of the bowel. This problem is referred to as *retention and overflow*. Sometimes (after about one to three weeks, when the rectum is so loaded that messages get through) a stool is let out when the child's muscle relaxes. The child usually doesn't realize that it is happening until it is too late. Some children, fearing ridicule or punishment, hide the evidence – the soiled clothing.

You will find different definitions of encopresis in textbooks. Because research suggests that soiling (and children who soil) cannot meaningfully be compartmentalized into disorders with physical, as opposed to psychological, aetiologies, or into any other recognizable groupings, a broad and simple definition will do: *a soiling child refers to any child over the age of four and under the age of 16 who regularly soils his/her underwear and/or bed.*

Some background information on encopresis

> It is not an uncommon problem. Three in every 100 children entering primary school at five years will still be soiling. Between

seven and eight years, about two out of 100 children are soiling. At 12 years, about one in every 100 boys (and some girls) are still soiling. Because of the shame felt about this problem, and the attempt by many families to keep the soiling a secret, the figures quoted may be underestimates.

➢ Constipation, or hard bowel movements, cause pain, irritability and a decreased appetite.

➢ A child's emotional state (due to stress/trauma) can affect the functioning of the bowel. Thus, soiling may result from distressing individual and/or family life-events such as sexual abuse (Boon, 1991).

➢ Many parents are likely to think (shamefully) that their child has a unique problem because most parents have never heard of another with a soiling problem.

➢ Some children have *never* established bowel control ('primary encopresis'). When bowel control has been established for at least six months before the soiling begins, it is referred to as 'secondary encopresis'.

➢ Soiling is not a unitary symptom, but a many-sided syndrome.

➢ For example, it can lead to fear, embarrassment and a lowering of self-esteem in the child, which lead on to yet other social ramifications. He or she is quite likely to be taunted, teased, even bullied at school because of the problem. (Children have been suspended from school because staff find soiling so difficult to manage.) For the family, there are feelings of bewilderment, frustration, failure, revulsion and anger. Soiling tends to engender negative responses from parents and is one of the most common precipitants of physical abuse incidents (see Claydon and Agnarsson, 1991).

➢ Soiling is sometimes associated with behaviour problems such as non-compliance and defiance.

➢ More boys soil than girls.

➢ Children of all levels of ability soil.

➢ Children from all walks of life soil.

➢ There is a highly significant association between enuresis and encopresis.

➢ There is a relationship between soiling and low birth weight.

➢ Children have to be taught to become clean, that is to say they have to be toilet-trained. It doesn't just happen!

There are three types of faecal soiling (see Hersov, 1994; Levine and Bakow, 1976):

1. where there is adequate bowel control but, nevertheless, the child deposits faeces in inappropriate places;
2. where there is a failure to gain bowel control; the child is unaware s/he is soiling or is aware but cannot do anything about it;
3. when the soiling is due to excessively fluid faeces.

Social learning theory

The previous point mentioned, that children must be taught to become clean, is of vital importance to interventions with soilers. Principles of learning and training (or re-training) strategies will be basic to our work. In all cultures bowel training is the responsibility of the mother, and most children have successfully learned bowel control between the ages of two and four, irrespective of the training methods used or how early they were applied. This guide does not deal, as its main emphasis, with early failures of training (that is, 'primary encopresis'). The point of the quotation at the beginning of this book is to highlight the complex social learning (the psychology) involved in the control and social response to an essentially physical activity (defecation). If this learning occurs under stress, it may break down under stress. Undue pressure (and this will apply to our training programmes) is the last thing in the world to facilitate learning!

Why do children soil?

Causation

There is no uniform causation for all cases of soiling; it comes about in different ways and for quite different reasons. Rigorous assessment is therefore crucial. The search for antecedent influences which may be linked with the problem produces a list of factors ranging from the intellectual (such as learning disability); the physical (for example, constipation); the psychological (fear of the toilet) or social (neglectful or coercive training in toilet habits).

Physical causes: constipation

The vast majority of cases of soiling are a result of chronic constipation and stool withholding. Not surprisingly, then, our particular interest in this manual is with *retention and overflow*. Children of any age who have hard movements (pain may also be caused by an anal fissure) may respond by stool withholding. When they feel the urge to have a bowel movement, they are afraid of experiencing pain and respond by holding the stool in. The role of the colon and rectum is to absorb water from the stool, so the longer the child withholds, whether voluntarily or involuntarily, the harder and more painful his/her bowel movements become. A 'vicious cycle' is created of stool withholding, causing more painful bowel movements, causing more stool withholding, and so on *ad nauseam*.

When the bowel is frequently overloaded, the rectal muscles become *overactive* while concurrently the anal muscles relax reflexly in response to the rectal activity (Clayden, 1988). Thus, as the muscles go on churning to eliminate the blockage, the child has no voluntary control over what happens below, and he/she soils. No wonder a child said to me, 'It's not me who soils, it's my bottom'. His bottom seemed to him to have an independent existence!

Other physical conditions

These include undiagnosed Hirschsprung's disease, intestinal obstructions, congenital abnormalities, gastrointestinal disease, brain injury and developmental delay, and can be read about in Clayden and Agnarsson (1991).

Psychological determinants

I have chosen the word 'determinants', rather than 'causes', deliberately, as the psychological factors associated with soiling may be secondary to the soiling – an 'emotional overlay' which *contributes* to the onset, maintenance or exacerbation of the symptoms. *Cause* is too precise a word.

Among the psychological determinants are:

➤ coercive training/punitive remedies on the part of parents;
➤ the role of anxious/overprotective mothers and overly strict fathers (Bellman, 1966);
➤ a tendency of soilers to be nervous (Bellman, 1966);
➤ a tendency of soilers to be food refusers (Bellman, 1966);
➤ a tendency of soilers to suffer from learned helplessness (Sluckin, 1981).

Environmental factors

Among the predisposing environmental influences are:

➤ stressful environments (Butler and Golding, 1986);
➤ poor toilets at home or at school;
➤ separation (and other traumatic) experiences;
➤ dietary factors: eating a diet deficient in fibre and drinking excessive milk can cause constipation in older children.

How to help soilers help themselves

The assessment

Points to remember:

➤ Parents and child are likely to be deeply embarrassed.
➤ You need a common language to discuss toileting and soiling issues with them. Most families have their own words (for example, loo, toilet, lavatory, potty; poohs, Number 2s, big jobs).
➤ The collaborative approach stresses the desirability of discovering what the child and his/her parents wish to do about the problem. Respect their views and give them time to express them.
➤ It also puts an emphasis on empowering the parents by providing them with knowledge and skills, and by sharing your thinking with them. Engage them in an active partnership during the assessment and (later) the intervention. One way of sharing information with parents is to give them the accompanying *Hints for Parents* and work through it with them. (Incidentally, sharing information reduces the number of clients who drop out of therapy, a particular problem in the case of soiling.)
➤ The assessment is not only about soiling; it is about a child with an embarrassing, restrictive problem; a child with feelings, and a child with a family who are also experiencing powerful emotions and attitudes about the child's 'failure'.

Steps for assessing the problem

Step 1. Ask for precise details of the soiling and any other behaviour problems.

Step 2. Use the ABC model and the Soiling Behaviour Checklist (both following) to systematize your data.

Step 3. Formulate hypotheses about the pattern of causes and determinants in this case of soiling (see Contributory Causes Checklist, p. 23).

THE ABC APPROACH TO ASSESSING BEHAVIOUR

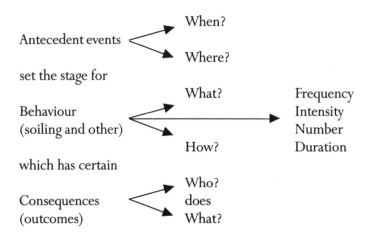

This fundamental analysis requires parental recording plus interview data based upon the following checklists (see Clayden and Agnarsson, 1991).

The Soiling Behaviour Checklist

➤ When is the child most likely to be soiled:
  at any time?
  morning?
  afternoon?
  night-time?
  in bed?
➤ Is the soiling problem a long-standing one?
➤ Are the motions normal in appearance and consistency?
➤ Does the child have a 'mass' of constipated motions?
➤ Does the child have diarrhoea?
➤ Does the child ever pass a motion in the toilet?
➤ Does the child hide when passing/having passed a motion?

> ➤ Do you assist the child with his/her toileting?
> ➤ Do you criticize when the child has soiled?
> ➤ Do you smack when the child has soiled?
> ➤ Are there *any* consequences when he/she soils?
> ➤ Do you feel your child soils frequently?
> ➤ Are there any other problems of behaviour you are worried about?
> ➤ Has your child had a recent medical examination for soiling?

Contributory Causes Checklist

	Yes	No	Detail

Are the following present:

Faecal masses (severe constipation)
Painful passing of motions
Fear of going to the toilet
Abnormal appearance/consistency of motions
Diarrhoea
Anal lesion/fissures
Failure to teach child bowel control
Stressful early bowel training (punitive,
    coercive, too early)
Unsatisfactory toilet arrangements
Inadequate/inappropriate diet
Stressful life events (at present)
Stressful life events (around time of
    onset of soiling)
Teasing/bullying at home or school
    in connection with soiling
Behaviour problems
High emotional arousal surrounding the
    bowel function (anger, resentment,
    despair, shame) at home
Abnormal response to bowel function
    (hiding, smearing, hiding underwear)
Refusal to go to sit on the toilet/sit on the potty
Defiance of a general kind (child)
Dysfunctional (parental attitudes overprotective,
    punitive, rejecting)
Abuse (physical/sexual/emotional)

Treatment

The intervention

Points to remember

➤ In this guide we are dealing mainly with the kind of soiling that involves retention with overflow.

➤ If you hear your mental alarm bells ringing because you have identified possible emotional or behavioural disturbance, seriously disruptive family dysfunction, developmental delay or child abuse, refer the family to a child and family consultation service or social services department.

The intervention has four strands to it:

1. **Medication**: laxatives are used to ensure effective rectal emptying and, eventually, the recovery of sensations related to defecation and continence.
2. **Food**: a high fibre diet helps to ensure continuance of rectal emptying.
3. **Routine**: routines are established to facilitate the timing of defecation and to establish toileting habits in the child.
4. **Training**: behavioural methods are used to facilitate the child's learning or relearning.

Medication

➤ Docusate and picosulphate are used to get rid of the old, hard stools by softening and 'dissolving' them. Enemas may have to be used in some cases.

➤ Medication is required to help send the stools along more quickly and make the rectum contract more. Senokot is commonly used for this purpose.

➤ There are medicines which provide roughage and keep the stools soft (for example Lactulose).

Food

➤ Some foods slow down the movement of the bowels (for example milk) or put the child off his/her food because they are filling (for example sweets).

➤ High fibre foods help to keep stools soft.

Routines

> ➤   The body requires routines (regular rhythms of eating, sleeping, passing a motion).
> ➤   The judicious use of senna, plus the routines prescribed in the behavioural programme, may provoke the passage of a stool at a time convenient for the child.

Training

This brings us to the use of behavioural programmes.

Preliminaries

(i)   If the child is fearful about going to the toilet/passing a motion, you will need to desensitize his/her fears (see Herbert, 1987).

(ii)   The child will find it hard to pass a motion if s/he is tense. You might suggest music, a comic, pictures or a toy to help them relax just so long as they are not distracted from the primary task.

(iii)   Children often need reminders to go and make an effort on the toilet. Parents *and* child may need reminders (such as a script, for keeping to the programme).

(iv)   Praise and encouragement and more tangible rewards (reinforcers) will facilitate learning and make the sometimes unpleasant toileting activity less burdensome for the child. Reward effort *and* success.

(v)   Before initiating the programme ensure that the constipation is under control; if not, failure will ensue.

(vi)   Remember: failure breeds failure; success breeds success.

The programme

The steps the programme might follow include:

(a)   Initiating the treatment plan on the basis of a *negotiated* working agreement.

(b)   Moving toward simple early goals, applying methods that are ethically acceptable and which have been explained to parents and accepted by them.

(c)   Collecting data as measures of change (for example ratings of behaviour, interactions, diary writing). A proforma 'My Chart' for recording soiling is at the back of the guide.

(d)   Using and interpreting data as a basis of monitoring.

(e)   Giving encouragement and fostering a positive approach.
(f)   Explaining that people may experience setbacks before making progress again.
(g)   Pinpointing particular difficulties.
(h)   Negotiating further goals if necessary.
(i)   Drawing upon the person's own ideas and motivation to indicate (and facilitate) progress.
(j)   Trouble-shooting promptly as difficulties arise.

The behavioural family therapy and behavioural parent training approaches require the therapist to be an energetic collaborator. To do this:

(a)   *Negotiate.* The key question is, 'How are we *together* going to address the problems?'
(b)   *Educate.* This involves the clarification of ideas about the soiling disorder and treatment. It means providing explanations, empowering parents by giving reasons, sharing information and increasing knowledge. It is helpful to mention examples of other people's success despite the difficulties.
(c)   *Observe.* Clients are encouraged and helped to observe their own (and their child's) reaction to the methods used and shown how to record them during treatment.
(d)   *Rehearse behaviour.* Clients are given the opportunity to practise, in an atmosphere where they feel comfortable and unthreatened, coping skills such as relaxation skills, self-talk and anger/impulse control and child management skills, for example, giving instructions and being consistent.
(e)   *Rehearse self-talk.* Clients are encouraged to rehearse positive 'coping statements' for example 'I can manage'; 'I can cope with this situation'; 'stay calm, breathe slowly, quietly'.
(f)   *Elicit support.* If necessary, and if the client permits, other members of the family or outside helpers are brought in as aides.
(g)   *Demythologize.* It is often necessary to counter the myths and attributions that get in the way of therapeutic change (for example, 'my child dirties himself as a way of getting at me').

An ethical rationale for using behavioural methods

The overall principles determining the choice of therapeutic methods are those of enhancing individual skills, reducing antisocial behaviour, alleviating personal distress, and (as a result) improving the quality of family life. The techniques chosen should always be used within an overall planned programme of management. There are also several ethical imperatives to be taken into account and fully discussed with parents.

The choice of methods

It is one of the strengths of behavioural work that treatment and the choice of methods do not depend necessarily upon the discovery and understanding of the historical causes of behaviour problems. The identification of the current problem and its contemporary antecedents and consequences is the main agenda in treatment. Very rarely can current problems be traced to specific past experiences with any degree of confidence.

Among the therapeutic tasks served by behavioural methods are the following:

➤ the acquisition (that is, the learning) of a desired response of which the individual is deficient, such as appropriate toileting behaviour, compliance, self-esteem, self-control.

➤ the reduction or elimination (the unlearning) of an unwanted response in the client's repertoire (such as self-depreciatory self-talk, aggression, temper tantrums, refusal to go to the toilet, hiding soiled underwear).

Explaining behavioural methods to parents

The application of behavioural methods to soiling (and other problems) depends, for their effectiveness, on a clear explanation of *what* is involved, and *why* they are thought likely to work (that is, their rationale). I suggest the following as one way of introducing these ideas.

Practitioner to parent: *Many of the problems of childhood are due not only to the child learning inappropriate (that is to say, undesirable) behaviours but the consequence of the child's failure to learn appropriate (in other words, acceptable, or socially desirable) behaviours and skills. Many problems in children, especially in the early years, are associated with inadequate skills involving self- or bodily-control. We shouldn't be too surprised as children are learners about life. It's a pity they don't wear figurative L plates to remind us of this fact! The word learning is the key idea here; indeed, it is the key to* *helping you and your child with his/her soiling. To do anything well demands good training; and involves two persons: a learner and a teacher. We need to teach your child useful toileting habits while training his/her body (that is to say, his/her bowel) to communicate more effectively with him/her by getting it back into good working order. You, as parents, will be wise guides and mentors.*

Acquiring/strengthening behaviour and skills

Method 1. Positive reinforcement

This method of intervention attempts to influence or control the outcome of certain prosocial behaviours or skills (for example, use of the toilet) through the use of positive reinforcers, that is, pleasurable consequences.

It is undoubtedly useful to begin with an explanation of positive reinforcement such as the following.

Practitioner to parent: *If the consequences of a behaviour are rewarding (that is, favourable) to a child, the behaviour is likely to increase in strength and it may become more frequent. Put another way: if the child does something like making an effort on the toilet, and as a result of this action something pleasant happens, then the child is more likely to do the same thing in similar circumstances in the future. When psychologists refer to this pleasant outcome as the positive reinforcement of behaviour, they have in mind several kinds of reinforcers: tangible rewards (such as extra TV/computer game time, treats, pocket money); social rewards (such as attention, a smile, a pat on the back, a word of encouragement); and self-reinforcers (that is, the ones that come from within and which are non-tangible, such as self-praise, self-approval, and a sense of pleasure or achievement.*

Questions to think through with parents

The following questions can help to generate training strategies.

Are you making good behaviour worthwhile?

Some parents remember to reward ('reinforce') desirable behaviour. The following examples could be printed on cards for you to use with them.

Antecedents	Behaviour	Consequences
Sandra was asked to tell her mother when she felt a pooh coming on.	She did so.	Her mum gave her a big hug and said 'good girl'.

> **Practitioner to parent**: *Sandra is likely to repeat this pattern. In order to improve or increase her performance of certain actions, you could think about how to arrange matters so that a reinforcing event (it might be an activity your child enjoys) follows the correct performance of toileting behaviour. You might indicate your intentions by saying, for example, 'When you have tried to do a pooh on the toilet then you can go out to play. I'll put a sticker on your chart: one for trying and one if you manage to do anything'. This is the useful 'when–then' rule.*

To have most effect, behavioural research shows that reinforcers such as treats, favoured activities, praise and encouragement, should follow as closely as possible upon the child's performance of the particular desired behaviour. Thus the parent who sensitively monitors their children and is quick to draw attention to success is likely to be using praise and encouragement more effectively than the parent who only gives favourable comments when, for example, the child does something quite extraordinary.

Are you making good behaviour unworthwhile?

Some parents persistently overlook or ignore their children's desirable actions:

Antecedents	Behaviour	Consequences
Philip's mother suggested he take himself to the toilet without prompting.	He did so.	Nil! Mother made no comments.

> **Practitioner to parent**: *It won't be surprising if Philip doesn't take himself to the toilet next time around. Do you perhaps fail to notice your child's good efforts?*

Method 2. Negative reinforcement

The initial description might go as follows:

> **Practitioner to parent**: *Behaving in a manner that avoids an unpleasant outcome leads to the reinforcement of behaviour, thus making*

it more likely to recur in similar circumstances. If your child does something you do not like, such as refusing to sit on the toilet as contracted in the behavioural programme, you may increase his/her ability to keep to the agreement by penalizing consistently (for example, the loss of TV time) for failing to do so. In this way you are providing what is called 'negative reinforcement' for his/her efforts to fulfil the agreed terms of the contract. You may not have to apply the penalty if s/he believes your threat because of your record for keeping your word. For example, if you say 'If you do not keep to what you agreed with Mrs. Brown I will not allow you to watch the television', then his/her resolve to think first and stick to the rules will be strengthened.

It is important to check on what is being asked of the child, and on what has or has not been taught them. Children can hardly be blamed for not doing what they don't know, are not capable of, or see to be unacceptable. The following questions are pertinent:

> Are the expectations of the child (skills, requirements) reasonable?
> Does he/she know *what* to do?
> Does he/she know *how* to do it?
> Does he/she know *when* to do it?

Of course, children may have been taught, and know, the socially appropriate behaviour or skills and when to produce them but still not perform them. So there are two more questions to ask:

> How can I get him/her to do what I want him/her to do?
> Now that he/she does it, how can I encourage him/her to continue doing it?

Parent to practitioner: *My trouble is that I'm on my own and I haven't always got the energy to insist on what I want her to do in following the programme. She is so defiant.*

Practitioner to parent: *Many parents tell us about this dilemma. You have to make a decision about a short-term investment of energy for long-term advantage. Your daughter plays off that side of you that is exhausted and wishes to take the 'line of least resistance' against that part that wishes to make a stand on an important matter of principle. If you can be firm and consistent for a week or two you'll find that your child will come to believe that you really mean what you say and will be more obedient. It's a costly, but profitable investment of your time and resolve.*

There is another important form of learning which it is important to convey to parents – observational learning, or less technically, imitation.

Method 3. Observational Learning (Modelling)

Practitioner to parent: *Children learn much of their social behaviour (and many other complex actions) by imitating others. They model themselves on their observations of the significant people in their environment, or symbolic figures, copying what they do and say. To teach a child new patterns of behaviour, give him or her the opportunity to observe a doll or puppet performing the desired actions of going to the toilet, passing a motion, cleaning itself and doing up its clothing.*

Method 4. Self-management training

In order to engender or strengthen self-control, change the child's instructions to him/herself (especially if the self-talk is negative: 'I'll never stop soiling'; 'I'm a big baby'). Training involves raising the client's consciousness of the circumstances in which s/he needs to go to the toilet; it then moves through a series of stages: first the therapist models the performance of a task, making appropriate and positive self-statements (for example, 'Think first, what is my body telling me?' 'It's telling me my bowel is full: I'll go to the toilet and see if I can pass a motion'). The client then practises the same behaviour, gradually moving to whispered, and eventually silent, self-instruction. Children are encouraged to use self-statements so that they can observe, evaluate and reinforce appropriate behaviours in themselves!

Behaviour problems

Soiling is sometimes accompanied by *behaviour problems*, many of which are attention-seeking strategies. The child learns that certain kinds of behaviour appear to attract parental attention, and in consequence, these forms of behaviour become part of their *habitual pattern* of behaving – what we call their *repertoire*. Because parents are often unaware of what is going on, they unwittingly but frequently reinforce in the child the very behaviours that they most wish to discourage. For example, they may reward children with attention every time they misbehave, and ignore them when they are co-operating.

Reducing behaviours that are undesirable

Method 5. Time-out from positive reinforcement (TO)

Time-out has been shown to be an effective penalty if taught as a disciplinary method to parents (Herbert, 1987). The procedure is intended to reduce the frequency of an undesirable behaviour by ensuring that it is followed by a reduction in the opportunity to acquire reinforcements, or rewards. In practice, we can choose from three forms of time-out.

1. *Activity time-out* where the child is simply barred from joining in an enjoyable activity but still allowed to observe it – for example, having misbehaved s/he is made to sit out of a game.
2. *Room time-out* where s/he is removed from an enjoyable activity, not allowed to observe this, but not totally isolated – for example standing at the far end of the sitting room.
3. *Seclusion time-out* where s/he is socially isolated in a non-frightening situation away from the reinforcing contingencies.

Time-out may last from three to five minutes. Always counterbalance TO with positive attention such as play, praise, additional contact for desirable behaviour. The best outcomes are obtained when both praise and time-out are employed.

Method 6. Response–cost

The use of response–cost procedures involves a penalty being invoked for failure to complete a desired response. This may involve the forfeiture of rewards currently available as, for example, when failure to sit on the toilet, as agreed, results in the loss of television privileges. It is a feature of the collaborative approach with this, as with other methods, that we ask parents to help us problem-solve our way through to solutions.

References

Anthony, E.J. (1957). An experimental approach to the psychopathology of childhood: Encopresis. *British Journal of Medical Psychology, 30,* 146–175.

Bellman, M. (1966). Studies in encopresis. *Acta Paediatrica Scandinavica (Suppl.), 170,* 7–132.

Boon, F. (1991) Encopresis and sexual assault. *Journal of the American Academy of Child and Adolescent Psychiatry, 30,* 479–482.

Butler, N. and Golding, M. (1986). *From Birth to Five: A Study of the Health and Behaviour of British Five Year Olds.* Oxford: Pergamon Press.

Clayden, G.S. (1988). Is constipation in childhood a neurodevelopmental abnormality? In P.J. Milla (Ed.) *Disorders of Gastrointestinal Motility in Childhood.* Chichester: Wiley.

Clayden, G.S. and Agnarsson, U. (1991). *Constipation in Childhood.* Oxford: Oxford University Press.

Devlin, J.B. and O'Cathain, C. (1990). Predicting treatment outcome in nocturnal enuresis. *Archives of Disease in Childhood, 65,* 1158–1161.

Doleys, D.M. (1977). Behavioural treatments for nocturnal enuresis in children: A review of the recent literature. *Psychological Bulletin, 84,* 30–54.

Dollard, J. and Miller, N.E. (1950). *Personality and Psychotherapy.* New York: McGraw-Hill.

Essen, J. and Peckham, C. (1976). Nocturnal enuresis in childhood. *Developmental Medicine and Child Neurology, 18,* 577–589.

Fergusson, D.M., Horwood, L.J. and Shannon, F.T. (1986). Factors related to the age of attainment of nocturnal bladder control: an 8-year longitudinal study. *Pediatrics, 78,* 884–890.

Halliday, S., Meadow, S.R., and Berg, I. (1987). Successful management of daytime enuresis using alarm procedures: a randomly controlled trial. *Archives of Disease in Childhood, 62,* 132–137.

Herbert. M. (1987). *Behavioural Treatment of Children with Problems: A Practical Manual.* London: Academic Press.

Hersov, L. (1994). Faecal soiling. In M. Rutter, E. Taylor, and L. Hersov (Eds) *Child and Adolescent Psychiatry: Modern Approaches* (3rd edn). Oxford: Blackwell Scientific Publishers.

Levine, M.D. and Bakow, H. (1976). Children with encopresis: a study of treatment outcome. *Paediatrics, 50,* 845–852.

Rutter, M., Tizard, J. and Whitmore, K. (Eds) (1970). *Education, Health and Behaviour.* Harlow: Longman.

Schmidt, B.D. (1986). New enuresis alarms: safe, successful and child operable. *Contemporary Pediatrics, 3,* 1–6.

Sears, R.R., Maccoby, E.E. and Lewin, H. (1957). *Patterns of Child Rearing.* London: Harper and Row.

Shaffer, D. (1994). Enuresis. In M. Rutter, E. Taylor and L. Hersov (Eds). *Child and Adolescent Psychiatry: Modern Approaches.* Oxford: Blackwell Scientific Publishers.

Sluckin, A. (1981). Behavioural social work with encopretics, their families and the school. *Child Care, Health and Development, 7,* 67–80.

Smith, P.S. and Smith, L.J. (1987). *Continence and Incontinence: Psychological Development and Treatment.* London: Croom Helm.

Tierney, A. (1973). Toilet training. *Nursing Times, 20/27 December,* 1740–45.

Webster-Stratton, C. and Herbert, M. (1994). *Troubled Families: Problem Children.* Chichester: Wiley.

Weir, K. (1982). Night and day wetting among a population of three year olds. *Developmental Medicine and Child Neurology, 24,* 479–484.

Further reading

Buchanan, A. (1992). *Children Who Soil.* Chichester: Wiley.

Herbert, M. (1993). *Working with Children and the Children Act.* Leicester: BPS Books (The British Psychological Society).

Morgan, R. (1981). *Childhood Incontinence: A Guide to Problems of Wetting and Soiling for Parents and Professionals.* London: Heinemann Medical Books Ltd.

Rutter, M., Yule, W. and Graham, P. (1973). Enuresis and behavioural deviance: some epidemiological considerations. In I. Kolvin, R.C. MacKeith, and S. Meadows (Eds). *Bladder Control and Enuresis*. Spastics International Medical Books Ltd.

Useful guides

For children
Eric's Wet to Dry Bedtime Book, Richard Butler. Published by Nottingham Rehab, 1989. A self-help manual for seven year olds and older.
You and Your Alarm, Jennifer Adams. Published by ERIC, 1990. A guide for children aged seven years and over on how to use the alarm or buzzer.

For parents
Your Child's Alarm, Jennifer Adams. Published by ERIC, 1990. A practical guide for parents to help their children use the alarm or buzzer.
A Guide for Parents, Penny Dobson. Published by ERIC, 1988 (reprint 1990). A twelve page guide giving tips on what parents and children can try and ways professionals can help children overcome bedwetting.

For professionals
A Guide to Enuresis, Christina Blackwell and Penny Dobson (Eds). Published by ERIC, 1989. A practical handbook for all professionals working with children with bedwetting and daytime problems. Adaptations of proformas from this excellent handbook and from my own practice are to be found at the back of this guide.

Enuresis Resource and Information Centre (ERIC), 65 St Michael's Hill, Bristol BS2 8DZ (0117 9 264 920)

Appendix I: A toilet training programme

Applications

> ➤ To establish regular use of the toilet.
> ➤ To re-establish toileting skills and muscular control after chronic constipation.

Caution

> ➤ There should be no element of coercion or punishment.
> ➤ If there is a behavioural problem of non-compliance it is crucial that the toilet itself doesn't become a battleground.
> ➤ Gradually hand over control of the programme to the child.

Procedure

> ➤ Obtain a medical check in case a mild laxative/bulking agent is required.
> ➤ Arrange for a warm drink at breakfast every morning.
> ➤ 15–20 minutes later, take the child to the toilet to attempt to pass a motion.
> ➤ Do not force the child to stay in the toilet longer than the five or so minutes necessary for the passing of a motion.
> ➤ Have a box for the child to rest his/her feet on. Encourage him/her to push (for example, pretend to be blowing up a balloon).
> ➤ Be aware of differing frequencies in individuals. Use baseline recordings (a diary) to determine whether the child has a bowel movement every day, every alternate day, or more than once a day, and adjust the programme accordingly.
> ➤ Continue supervised regular toileting until the child has established appropriate defecation for two weeks. This means taking the child to the toilet, prompting the child to go to the toilet, expecting self-initiated toileting and prompting the child when this is not forthcoming.
> ➤ The handing over of responsibility to the child is vital (the aim of

routine training is to develop the child's awareness of the sensations and actions associated with appropriate use of the toilet).

➤   Provide rewards (praise, and, later, a tangible incentive) for *effort* as well as *success!*

Note

If the child is afraid to go to the toilet, reduce his/her anxiety by having the child gradually approach the toilet, taking the process in very small steps. This is a desensitization procedure.

➤   Start at a distance from the toilet at which the child is happy (even if this is halfway down the hall).
➤   Simply bring the child a little closer to the toilet.
➤   At each step towards the toilet, praise the child and give some tangible reward such as a piece of fruit or biscuit.
➤   Do NOT coerce the child. Stop when s/he becomes too anxious for the rewards to be pleasurable.
➤   Repeat the procedure three times a day until the child is able to sit comfortably on the toilet.

Appendix II: Designing the individual's programme

Every child is an individual, and unique. So is his/her family. Bowel movements are also individual; there are considerable variations in the need to defecate. Bowel movement can occur in healthy children several times a day, several times a week, or only a few times a month. Even the child's constipation has its individuality; each soiling problem is made up of its own particular mixture of predisposing causes, contributory precipitating influences, and social consequences. This means that there is no one behaviour formula, no set-pace programme to fit all cases. Each soiling programme needs to be individually designed, discussed and negotiated with the family. It is vital to involve the parent(s) *and* child in all aspects of the work.

The author discusses the design of programmes in detail elsewhere (see Herbert, 1987; 1993). However, it may be helpful to see the 'script' (usually typed out for parents) of a fairly typical kind of programme.

Example Script: PETER'S PROGRAMME
Organizer: Peter's mother, Sally Brown
Helper: School nurse, Mary Smith

Now that Peter's constipation has been cleared the agreement is to carry out the following plan that we have jointly agreed:
1.   To keep a record in the event diary of:
     (a)   his medication
     (b)   his going to the toilet and the results.
2.   Peter will have a hot drink with each meal (his diet has been discussed).
3.   Because the most likely time to be successful is after eating, he will go to the toilet about 15 minutes after each meal.
4.   Peter will sit there for at least 5 minutes. There will be some comics and his Walkman to keep him amused. However, he has promised:
     (a)   to try pushing, every so often, imagining (as we have practised) that he is blowing a balloon;

(b)   he will have a box to rest his feet on to help with the pushing;

(c)   even if he passes a small stool, he will go on trying, off and on, to pass yet another.

5.   *Incentives.* Peter's reward for co-operating so well and helping himself will be:

(a)   a happy face for his merit book for trying (and staying the full 5 minutes);

(b)   a further *two* happy faces sticker for producing a pooh.

6.   The family will look at Peter's charts and offer him encouragement (never criticism) and praise for trying.

7.   When Peter has collected X happy faces his mum and dad will take him to Y for a treat.

8.   Mrs. Smith will stay in touch and review the progress of the programme in Z days/weeks.

Appendix III: Daytime Record Chart

Award a sticker for: (1) emptying bladder in toilet.
(2) holding on.

Fill in a new line for EACH VISIT to the toilet.

Name: .... Week beginning: ....

Date	Put a sticker on for a visit to the toilet	Time of day	Did you need to go? N – not urgently U – urgently E – extremely urgently	Put a sticker on for holding on	How long did you hold on for?

Appendix IV: Baseline Night Record Sheet

Please check whether the bed is wet or dry:
(1) before going to bed yourself.
(2) in the morning.
Put W if wet and D if dry

	Week 1			Week 2	
	Night	Morning		Night	Morning
Monday					
Tuesday					
Wednesday					
Thursday					
Friday					
Saturday					
Sunday					

Appendix V: 'My Chart'

Name:

	Day 1	Day 2	Day 3	Day 4	Day 5	Day 6	Day 7
Week							

No soiling ☺

S for Soiled
(time noticed)

	Day 1	Day 2	Day 3	Day 4	Day 5	Day 6	Day 7
Week							

No soiling ☺

S for Soiled
(time noticed)

	Day 1	Day 2	Day 3	Day 4	Day 5	Day 6	Day 7
Week							

No soiling ☺

S for Soiled
(time noticed)

	Day 1	Day 2	Day 3	Day 4	Day 5	Day 6	Day 7
Week							

No soiling ☺

S for Soiled
(time noticed)

	Day 1	Day 2	Day 3	Day 4	Day 5	Day 6	Day 7
Week							

No soiling ☺

S for Soiled
(time noticed)

	Day 1	Day 2	Day 3	Day 4	Day 5	Day 6	Day 7
Week							

No soiling ☺

S for Soiled
(time noticed)

Draw a happy face in one square every morning before breakfast if I haven't soiled.
Put an S in the square, and the time, if I have an accident.

Appendix VI: A Colouring-In Incentive Chart

Colour in a child each time you are successful.

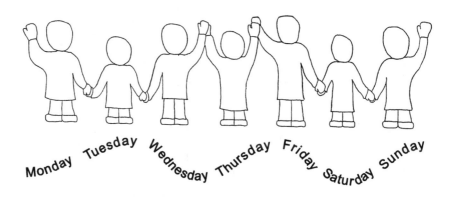

Monday   Tuesday   Wednesday   Thursday   Friday   Saturday   Sunday

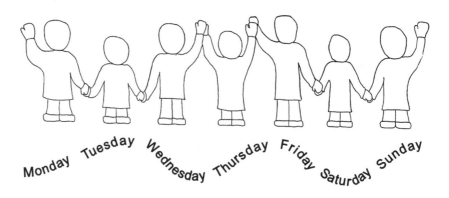

Monday   Tuesday   Wednesday   Thursday   Friday   Saturday   Sunday

Appendix VII: Treatment Record Sheet

Name: ....

In the first column, write a 'W' if the child was wet at all during the night, a 'D' if he or she was completely dry.

Night	W or D	Time of wetting	Patch size (small/medium/large)	Did the alarm wake the child?	Did the child wake without the alarm to use the toilet during the night?
Monday					
Tuesday					
Wednesday					
Thursday					
Friday					
Saturday					
Sunday					

Hints for Parents 1: Potty training

➤ Active training is most effective when the child is ready (generally between 18 and 24 months, probably nearer the latter).

➤ There is no one right way of training.

➤ Don't make a fuss; be matter of fact, for example discuss when changing nappies with the child what they've done, and what you are doing about it. Do the same when s/he toddles after you into the toilet when you are using it.

➤ Will training impose any emotional stress on the child? Not if you don't put undue pressure on him/her! You know your child and how best to pace the training process. Remember there may be vulnerable times, such as after an illness or separation when learning a new and difficult skill will be more difficult.

➤ Be prepared for setbacks: it is like learning to ride a bicycle. There may be wobbles, falls and other setbacks before becoming confident and perfect in riding performance.

The early steps can be facilitated by:

➤ anticipating the child who is regular (sitting him/her on the potty at the expected time or when the telltale signs (e.g. a red face) are visible);

➤ making a sit-on-the-pot part of the morning routine (before dressing) and evening routines (at bedtime);

➤ praising success (and effort);

➤ gradually increasing the frequency of sessions on the potty (avoid force and overlong and boring 'sittings');

➤ encouraging the child to let caregivers know when s/he has urinated or passed a bowel motion. The awareness of *having* wet or soiled precedes the awareness of *impending* urination or bowel movement!

➤ eventually leaving off nappies;

➤ teaching the child to help (and eventually manage) putting on and taking off of pants;

➤ reminding the child to ask for the potty – this means having it handy as there may be a rush to sit him/her on it;

➤ making liberal use of praise and encouragement for trying and success; avoid criticism and punishment;

> moving on eventually to the toilet, adapted for his/her use. (A step may be needed to help them reach.)

Bladder training

At eighteen months of age most children are physically mature enough to hold their urine for between one and two hours without much leakage. Their co-ordination, being able to sit comfortably on the potty or toilet, for example, would be another sign of readiness. Also their ability to understand simple instructions. Potty training might take a reasonably short time if your child is ready. Remember there are large individual differences in this readiness! The association between voluntarily passing urine and sitting on the potty should be made relatively easily if you remember to pot your child regularly. In the first few weeks it is up to you to anticipate her/his need and suggest sitting on the potty. Keep the training 'low key' and praise success.

In many instances it will not be necessary to make a special effort to train your child to control her/his bowels and to use the potty. S/he will automatically learn of this by passing a motion while doing a wee. It is important not to engender fear, embarrassment or shame if it does become necessary to institute training. Calm, matter-of-fact association of potty and passing a motion (by regular potting) should do the trick. Perceptive parents can 'read' the child's need to go to the toilet.

Hints for Parents 2: Problems of incontinence in children

That feeling of isolation

Parents often feel that only *their* child wets the bed/soils and that no one else knows what it is like not to have a dry/clean child. In fact, many do, but they tend to keep quiet about it.

What is bedwetting (enuresis)?

➢ the repeated, involuntary urinating during sleep

Clinicians are reluctant to use these technical terms (enuresis and encopresis) to denote a problem of incontinence until the child is over the age of five and four respectively. Both problems frequently occur in the same child.

Who wets/soils?

➢ Children from all walks of life
➢ Bright and not-so-bright children
➢ More boys than girls

Why do children wet/soil?

They do so for many reasons. The following are but a few:
➢ some have a physical condition that needs attention (e.g. a bladder infection/constipation);
➢ some have never learnt to use the toilet;
➢ some are reacting to stress;
➢ some need reminders, incentives or some other encouragement;
➢ some are immature, developmentally delayed;
➢ some are confused about what to do, or (perhaps) afraid of the toilet.

What can I do to help?

This depends on why your child wets/soils. The clinician will carry out an assessment and discuss the results with you; also a programme to help the child learn control. Research tells us that parents are the best ones to help children to get things right. A partnership between yourself, your child and the clinician is the best way forward.

Hints for Parents 3: Instructions for the use of the enuresis alarm

- ➤ While using the alarm, the child should sleep naked below the waist. The reason for this is that pyjama trousers or long nightdresses tend to absorb urine and thus delay triggering off the alarm; research evidence suggests that therapeutic effectiveness depends upon rapid triggering once wetting has commenced.
- ➤ When the alarm is triggered during the night, the child is required to switch the alarm off as rapidly as possible, and then complete urination in the toilet before returning to bed.
- ➤ While the alarm is in use, you should desist from 'lifting' – that is, awakening the child to urinate when the alarm has not been triggered, and imposing any restrictions on the child's fluid intake – a child under treatment should be permitted to drink whenever s/he wishes.
- ➤ You should ensure that the alarm is in use and switched on each night. The alarm should be used every night unless there are special circumstances rendering its use inappropriate (for example, when there are overnight visitors in the house, or when the child is away from home).
- ➤ Treatment records should be maintained on a chart. It is vital to the evaluation of progress that accurate and up-to-date records are kept.
- ➤ When the alarm has been triggered, you need to assist the child as necessary in waking, switching the alarm off, and visiting the toilet. Where the alarm alone fails to waken the child, you should first waken the child *while the alarm continues to sound*, encouraging the child to switch it off him/herself, guiding her/his hand as necessary, and only switching off for the child if s/he appears too unaware of events to do so. You should not switch the alarm off before waking the child, as this precludes association between waking and the sound of the alarm.
- ➤ The bed should be remade with dry bedclothing, the detector mats and waterproof sheets dried (a dry corner of the wet sheet is useful for this purpose), and the alarm reset in case of a second wetting incident. Depending upon age, your child may take responsibility for this task. Where the therapist judges the resetting of the

apparatus to be excessively burdensome (or bedlinen is particularly scarce), it may be omitted, particularly if the patient rarely wets more than once per night. Where a child wets more than once per night, it is however worth persevering in resetting the apparatus if possible, since multiple wetting usually reduces to one incident per night within two to three weeks of treatment by this.

(Note: wet sheets must be properly laundered before re-use, and not merely allowed to dry out, otherwise false alarm triggerings resulting from perspiration will be rendered more likely.)

Explanation of the treatment

The basis of alarm treatment is a process of learning, and thus each alarm triggering may be regarded as a lesson in bladder control.

It is important to appreciate that the enuresis alarm is not a 'magic box' which can be expected to terminate enuresis from the first night of its use, and that marked changes in the number of wet nights experienced often do not occur during the first month of treatment. It should also be noted that the progress of learning is rarely steady, but may be expected to include setbacks as it advances.

Explaining to the child

'When you have a wet night, what happens is that the tank for wee inside you, called your bladder, gets full and sends a message to your brain saying that it needs to be emptied. Your brain, though, is too sleepy to take any notice, so your bladder just has to empty in your bed and you have a wet night. When you are using the alarm, the buzzer wakes you up and stops you wetting as soon as this happens. After a while, your brain gets so used to being woken up just after it gets that message saying that your bladder is full, that instead of staying sleepy it learns to listen to what your bladder is saying, and either wakes you up in time to go to the toilet or tells you to hold on for a while.'

Hints for Parents 4: An explanation of bowel function for your child

This is a picture of what happens to the food you eat. When you swallow food, it goes through a long tube which winds around and around in your tummy. You need most of the food you eat to make you grow and keep you strong and healthy, but some of the food isn't needed, and this is squeezed along to the end of the tube in your tummy by your muscles. Just like squeezing toothpaste along to the end of the toothpaste tube. When the pooh gets to the end of the tube in your tummy, a message is sent to your brain saying: 'I need a pooh, I should go to the toilet'; and a message is sent to the muscles in your bottom saying: 'Time to open up and squeeze the pooh out'.

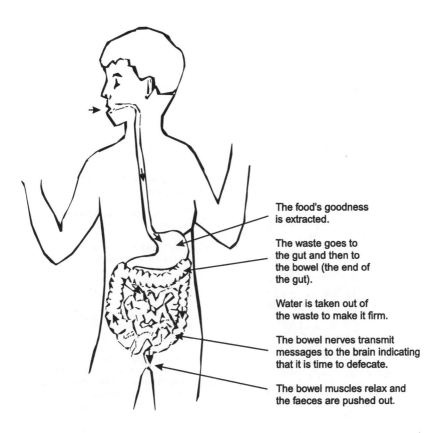

The food's goodness is extracted.

The waste goes to the gut and then to the bowel (the end of the gut).

Water is taken out of the waste to make it firm.

The bowel nerves transmit messages to the brain indicating that it is time to defecate.

The bowel muscles relax and the faeces are pushed out.

Hints for Parents 5: An explanation of soiling for your child

If you don't go to the toilet when your brain tells you, then more and more pooh collects at the end of the tube in your tummy and you can't get it out properly because there's too much, and it hurts. So to help you get it out, you need to see the doctor, who will give you some medicine to get all the pooh out so that the tube in your tummy will be all nice and unblocked again.

To stop pooh collecting at the end of the tube in your tummy, you have to get your muscles working hard again, so that they push your food along the tube in your tummy and open up to let the pooh out.

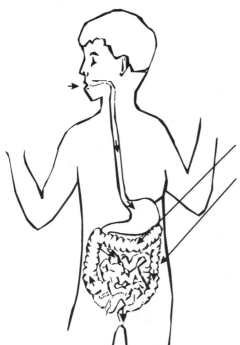

The waste is in the bowel for a long time.

The bowel nerves fail to send messages to the brain.

The child does not know that s/he needs to defecate.

Some faeces get pushed out on their own.

The waste remains in the bowel longer. Water is removed from the waste, which becomes very hard.

The hard waste is like small pieces of rock. The water waste leaks out around the hard faecal matter ('retention with overflow'). The child has no control over this.